Leaving With Love

Eternal Messages from the Heart

Gayla Gabriel

A Keepsake of Personal Notes
For Your Loved Ones

Gayla Gabriel

Published by Sparks of Light Publishing – Palos Verdes Peninsula, California

www.leavingwithlove.com
leavingwithlove@yahoo.com

ISBN-978-0-9801522-0-3

First edition printing December 2007

Cover photography by Janis Kerr. Cover design by Anthony L. Brown.

Printed in the USA

Dear Gayla,

Thanks for being there as a friend. You know, a long time ago I learned that the things in life that are most important can never be taken away – like our values, dignity, sense of well-being; but most importantly our true friends – friends like you.

God bless you.
I'll always love you.

Sonny

In Loving Memory
to
Sonny

Acknowledgements

Through this illuminating process of authoring and publishing this book, I learned there are sparks of light in everything we encounter in life, both human and nonhuman. Thus, I named my publishing company Sparks of Light. As this book developed, grew, and finally was born, my sense of these sparks of light heightened my appreciation for everything and everyone that became part of this process. My gratitude and appreciation goes deeper than just mentioning the following people who believed in this project and helped me bring it to its physical form; however, I wanted to mention them individually.

First, my son Jeremy, I love you, I love you . . . you are the best son a mother could have ever wished for all in one lifetime. Your continual encouragement and belief in my vision has truly been a gift. Thank you for always making me proud.

Anthony L. Brown, the book's art director and so much more! Thank you for your years of constantly assisting me in making choices and bringing this book alive as you formatted it onto paper and beyond!

Janet Carnay, loving friend, thank you for hours of listening to my concerns, editing, and contributing your beautiful photographs to this project. You have been a loving inspiration! I realize that as someone who experienced an unexpected and tragic loss you know the potential impact this book will have on loved ones.

Janis Kerr, thank you for your foresight in sharing your amazing photograph of the sky that became the backdrop for the dust cover and being a friend who has seen me through many of life's ups and downs.

Jeff Shulkin, my brilliant and caring friend, thank you for appearing when I needed your experienced voice. Graciously you shared your unique ideas that became a part of this project. As a widower you sensed the importance of this work. Your support helped keep me going!

Kathleen White, friend and former co-worker, your support and help at the infancy of this project was invaluable as the springboard that catapulted me forward.

Ned Mansour, thank you for taking an interest in this project, as a new friend, quiet advisor, and author of several books. Thank you for sharing your experience of writing a letter to loved ones and then sharing excerpts from it for the eulogy at a funeral. Your story touched me and made me feel that this book will touch the lives of many.

Several other notes of appreciation and gratitude for those that helped shape the manuscript with their critical eyes, contributions, and suggestions: Jim and Joanne Leth, Gus and Vivien Gallup, Judy Garvey, Jane McMannes, Jerry Sheby, Denyce Giannioses, and Art Keenan.

Please forgive me if I left anyone out this time around.

My gratitude to all those who are no longer here, but guided me with their whispers, and of course I owe everything to my constant partner . . . the Light.

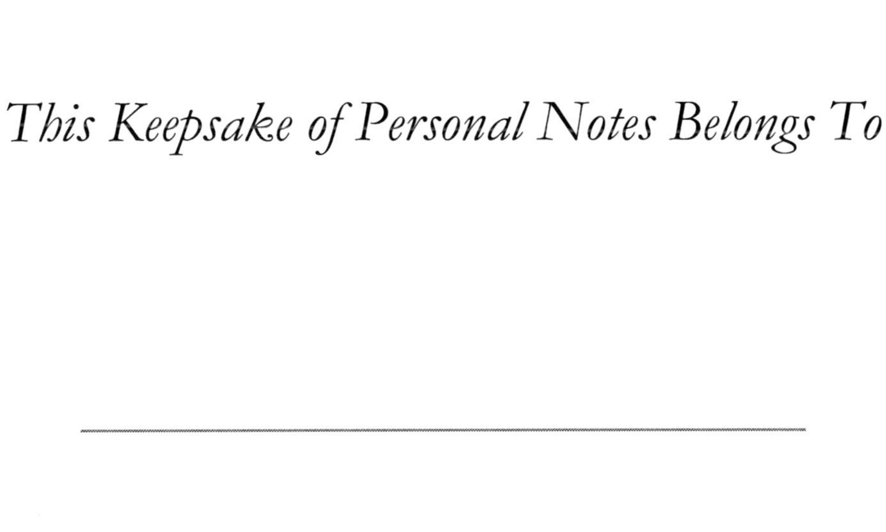
This Keepsake of Personal Notes Belongs To

Where Is The Table Of Contents?

As my dear friend Jeff Shulkin reviewed this book, I proposed excluding a conventional Table of Contents. He quickly responded by suggesting I call it Table of "Contentments." He felt as each section of the book was completed; slowly transforming the "book" into a Keepsake, there would also be personal transformation leading to contentment as one shares his or her love.

With that said, here you will see the order in which the book unfolds:

Purpose

Death is the one event in the changing nature of life that is inevitable. Fortunately, love is the one thing death cannot take with it. This book that transforms into a keepsake was created to give you an opportunity to leave more love behind for all the special people in your life and all the ones you have shared love with throughout your life. By using this keepsake as a vehicle for sharing your love, potentially you can become immortal through your messages, letters, notes and personal information. Initially, this project was originally conceived as I was experiencing my own personal heartbreak and loss. In the process of working through my own grief, working with other grievers as a grief counselor and witnessing many world tragedies, the importance and purpose for this book developed.

It is not until we are personally touched by loss or a major tragedy that we are forced to feel pain and the void left by the loss. Thus, we have been called a death-denying society. However, September 11, 2001 created a monumental shift in the attitude of millions of people. We were shocked into having a new relationship with loss. We are now more conscious about the truth that none of us know when or how we may leave this world. Today, it is difficult to deny the impermanence of life.

Engaging in the exercises throughout this book offers an amazing possibility to discover more about your personal gifts, talents, strengths, values, joys, wishes and more. My desire is to encourage you to think about the loved ones you will one day leave behind. Writing your heartfelt messages, you will leave an everlasting and intimate gift that will become a stepping stone for those you love, allowing them to move forward to the fulfillment of their own lives. Your eternal messages will allow you to leave with love.

Leaving With Love

It has been said that there is magic in the telling of a story. It is my hope that my story will empower you, as well as encourage you, to do something wonderful for those you love, by choosing to Leave with Love.

Valentine's Day had just ended. I was alone in my small apartment when the phone rang. My mother's voice, coming through the receiver, was telling me something I refused to comprehend. "How could he do this, I was just getting to know him! Are you sure? No, it can't be true!" My father was dead! Impossible! It was Valentine's Day. My dad and I had enjoyed lunch together at a local restaurant. I spoke to him a few hours later on the phone to get one of his favorite recipes.

Now he was gone! Our relationship of father and daughter was just starting to take form. I was nineteen and finally getting a sense of who my dad was, when unexpectedly, a sudden and massive heart attack claimed his life.

My father's sudden death left me feeling angry, abandoned, and betrayed for many years, because I realized with his sudden death I lost my chance to know more about my dad. What did he really think and feel about himself, his life, about my siblings, the world, and me? What dreams did he still have for his life? What hopes did he have for me, my sister and brother? How did he view his own life? What values did he still want to impart to me? I wanted to know so much more about my dad, about his heart, his soul, his very being. Bottom line was I wanted more of him – something from him I could hold on to and cherish. The final time I saw him, his last words were "I love you." For years I suffered, not knowing how to heal this huge void in my life, created by my father's unexpected death.

My father's passing was the unconscious seed for the writing of this book, which became clear to me in 1996. This was the year Sonny, a wonderful friend I had known for twenty-eight years, died from a brain tumor at age forty-eight.

Sitting in the chapel during Sonny's funeral, I looked around at the other people; there was a mix of friends and family. At that moment, I realized I had actually met Sonny at my father's funeral only steps away from this setting. This remembrance moved me to tears. I took out a piece of paper to write down a few of my thoughts and feelings about my dear friend, with the hopes of sharing them with all the people in attendance. The service began and the rabbi spoke for a few moments about Sonny, recalling the obvious to all of us: his kindness, generosity, and excellence in his work, along with other comments that could have been said about almost anyone. As I listened and waited, I was hoping that the rabbi conducting the service would invite others to share something personal about Sonny. I felt disappointed that nothing during the service reflected Sonny's personal passions. The music, the flowers, the verses read, and the absence of personal reflections usually shared by family or friends made this funeral quite generic for a man that had shared his life and his love in many unique and extraordinary ways.

Feeling empty and sad after Sonny's funeral, I realized that I needed and wanted more from this service. It became acutely clear to me that I was experiencing the same void I had felt since my father's death. Now I became conscious of the need to find a way to heal. I looked around and realized there were many people feeling the pain of Sonny's death. I had an enormous desire to reach out and ease the pain of his family members and friends as I empathized with their deep personal loss and grief. On my drive to the home of Sonny's brother, after the funeral, I started to envision the idea for this book.

A few weeks after Sonny's death, I lost my favorite uncle to cancer. Married fifty years to my uncle, my aunt found the loss of her partner extremely difficult. I remember speaking with my aunt before my uncle died. Several weeks before his death he chose to no longer communicate with my aunt verbally, so I suggested that she write him a love letter. She said it would make him cry and she didn't want to do that to him. After his funeral, while conversing with my aunt, she confessed that while packing my uncle's things, she was secretly hoping to find a letter from him. She never found one – no final love letter, no good-bye note, nothing. She was quite disappointed; even after more than fifty years of marriage, the need for one last communication of love prevailed!

These personal short stories, and several other stories I share later in the book, helped confirm to me that my idea for this manuscript made sense. My hope is that this book with its stories and heartfelt exercises will be a catalyst, a springboard for creating and sharing a wonderful keepsake of eternal messages for those you love. Allow yourself to feel the love, courage and compassion that will help you put your personal fears aside about death and dying. I believe if my father had left me a note or message my pain and grief might have been easier to bear.

Planning for your final rite of passage is one of the greatest gifts you can give your family, loved ones, and friends. As you embrace some of the many ideas and opportunities found within this book, it may become a catalyst for your own personal introspective process. Perhaps you will find yourself willing to share more of the real you and your feelings, beliefs, wishes, fears, talents, strengths, and love.

As you engage in the process of completing the exercises in this book, allow your emotions to flow so you can express your feelings and touch the hearts of those you love. My greatest hope is that this keepsake will ease the pain of your loved ones and be an everlasting gift for them designed by and sealed with your personal signature.

Personal Eternal Messages

Several summers ago, my cousin and I were having a lovely, leisurely lunch. As we slowly ate the delicious café food, I shared my idea for this book.

Her first response to the idea was not favorable. She couldn't see the purpose for preparing something to leave behind for those you love. I felt disappointed, but I listened to her reasons while I continued to enjoy my lunch. A few moments passed. Then my cousin broke the silence. Her voice became strained and cracking; I noticed tears welling up in her eyes.

My cousin, an only child, was extremely close to her parents. She had recently lost her father to a sudden heart attack and then her mom to cancer. She slowly described those two events. Holding back the tears, she told me that when her mom died she went to her parents' home to prepare it to be leased. My cousin told me that she found herself looking everywhere for a letter addressed to her from her dad. He was her favorite member in the family. Her disappointment in not finding a special note or letter was clearly written on her face as she quietly wept.

This experience of deep disappointment does not need to happen to someone you love. Consider leaving behind something special they can cherish. Writing special notes or letters to loved ones or special friends can become eternal gifts. They will be sacred and develop a life of their own.

As of late, we have all witnessed the tragedy of 9/11 and the ongoing wars. Story after story has focused on loved ones looking for personal keepsakes left by their loved ones. Survivors need and desire one final message. Even sound bites of phone messages left for them or heard by operators are still being listened to or sought from 9/11.

Today, soldiers are making videos for their families only to be viewed if they do not return. Recently, trapped miners wrote messages of love and hope on their own bodies, so they might convey their last messages of love. Do not wait! Convey your feelings to those special people now.

Give yourself time to sit and feel the love you have for each individual person. Be real. Be conscious of the process. You might even describe a few memorable times you shared together and what it meant to you then and now. Maybe you can share something valuable that you learned from their presence in your life. Like the excerpt from the lyrics to the song, "For Good," by Stephen Schwartz from the musical "Wicked," expressed so eloquently, "It well may be that we will never meet again in this lifetime so let me say before we part, so much of me is made of what I learned from you."

Doing this on audio tape, video or DVD is an option if you are not comfortable writing your thoughts.

As part of a loved one's grieving process, these eternal letters or messages will gently help them to open to their own future, without you.

As the idea for this book unfolded, I shared my thoughts with a few friends. My friend Jane, like my cousin, was not sure she could encourage me. Then she remembered reading Erma Bombeck's book, Motherhood, the Second Oldest Profession. Jane sent me the book and admitted that every time she read the chapter entitled "Julie" she cries. I cry, too.

It is a tender story about a young mother in her forties dying from cancer. Her three sons are unaware of her illness until her death when each is given a personal love letter from their mother, Julie. Each letter shares poignant moments from the son's birth and throughout his life that tell a loving story straight from the mother's heart.

When I shared the excerpt from Erma Bombeck's book with friends there were several responses.* One friend was inspired to write a letter of appreciation and gratitude to his aging parents. Another friend enrolled in a class that encouraged writing letters, sharing memoirs and personal feelings. Still another friend composed a letter to her daughter and a father composes letters on special days for his kids. Another poignant letter was written by a father after he woke up in the middle of the night, needing to share his loving thoughts with his daughter. With permission, I have included a few of these letters for you to read. May the beautiful messages of these letters inspire you to write your own personal eternal messages of love.

You may consider using your own stationery for writing these letters. Store them in the envelope provided so they will be found by your loved ones or share them now.

Motherhood, the Second Oldest Profession

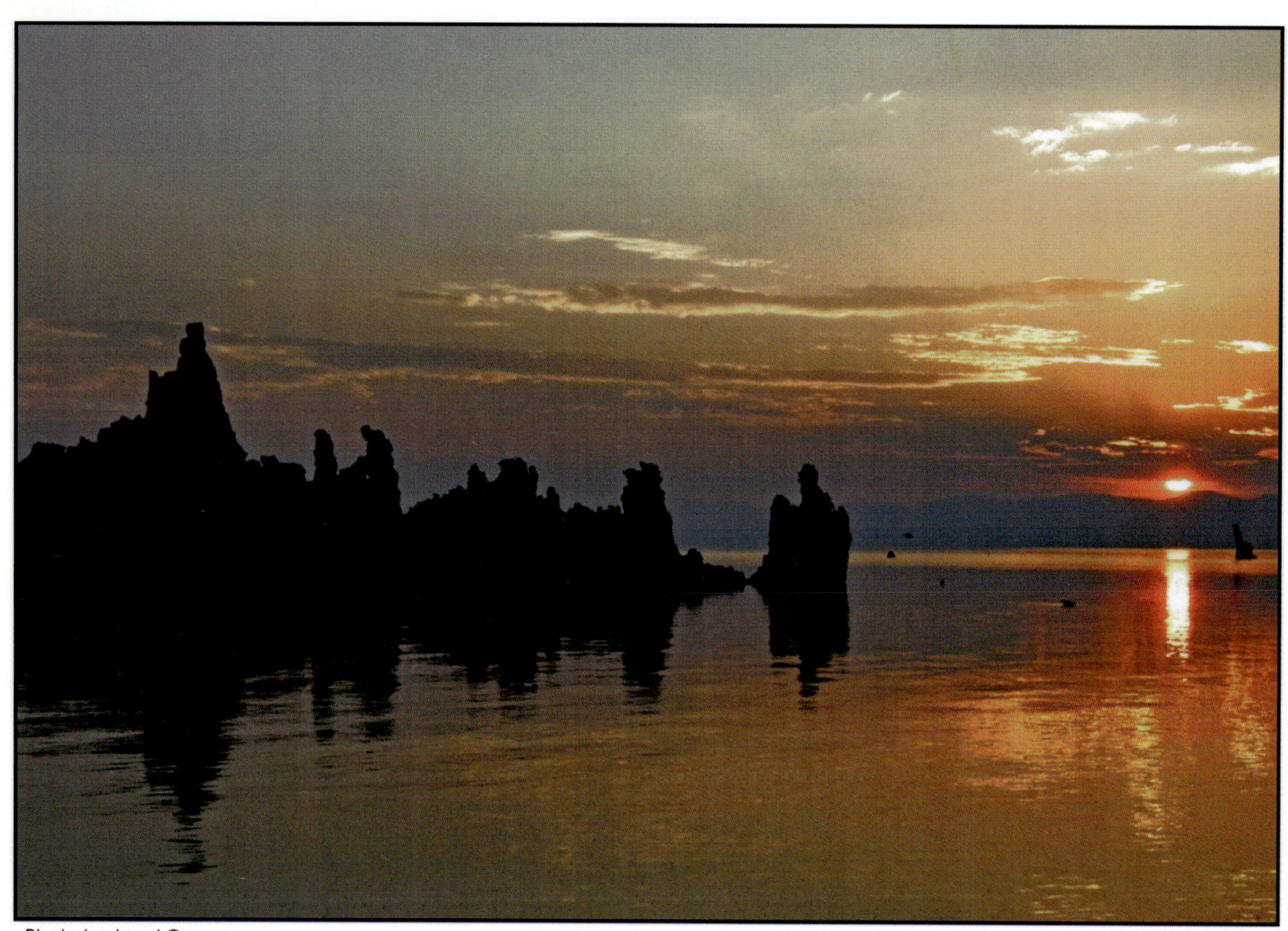

Photo by Janet Carnay

The First Letter

It was very early this morning when I awoke. My immediate thoughts were on you. Then I noticed tears on my pillow. What's this? Tears of joy or tears of compassion? Both, but more when I realized that my entire being was reaching out to you. It was a yearning to hold my little girl again; to comfort, to "make it go away, daddy." We have grown beyond that, and now you have your own to comfort. Just the same, the well from which these feelings flow never changes.

You have been deeply affected by things beyond your control, and things you cannot change. I would like to "make them go away." Even if I could, we both know that would be of no help to your growth.

Lately I have sensed a hard edge about you in response to the pressures on you. It reminds me that you are a fighter. It also reminds me that your father could "rise up in righteous indignation" at the drop of a hat. How far does the apple fall from the tree? Not as critic, but one who understands, it is OK to show your soft side at times. It is OK to be vulnerable.

I have known many people who have been thoughtful or kind or loyal or demonstrative in showing love and concern. I have known very few who are the complete package. You come closer than anyone I know. You will be truly blessed if your daughters mature to bring you the joy that you give me.

We all are so busy that we miss opportunities to hold one another. It's funny, as I grow older I see this: I held my children, I don't get to hold my grandchildren often enough, and now, I hold my dog and my cat.

Know this my chickadee, you may not be able to curl up in my lap, but you are securely curled in my heart and soul . . . forever.

The Second Letter

To My Dearest Daughter:

What does one say to the firstborn?

Suddenly I was a mother and parent and didn't have the slightest idea how to do that.

Like most mothers during that time we had Dr Spock's words of wisdom, but he didn't address the everyday decisions that had to be made when one has the total responsibility of caring for an infant.

Anyway, I was so busy trying to be a good mother that it was a while before I realized how much I had grown to love you.

I have learned in the years raising you that our children are ours for a short time and that they are here to teach us who they are.

Despite the many mistakes I made along the way I can reflect an all that you are and feel blessed to have had the time with you to learn who you are.

I found out that you are what I call an earth-mother. You are a person who is well rounded; who creates the space around her with beauty and love.

I also see you as a person who stands tall and is able to tell her truth.

You have strength, wisdom and inner beauty.

I once heard a commentator ask the question: Does the true character of a person show up when challenged because it is already there within or does one's character show up because of the challenge?

From the way you live your life I feel that the person that you are within meets the many challenges that you have faced because of your beautiful inner life.

Thank you for the honor and privilege of knowing and loving you.

With Love – Mom

The Third Letter

Kirk, another year has passed and it is summer. This has been an interesting year. Before I get started there are three things I want you to know and I never want to stop telling you.

- *How much I LOVE you. I know I have told you that before and you have told me you know it, but I don't ever want to stop telling you that I LOVE you. I don't think I tell you enough. I don't think I express my true feelings to you enough.*

- *How PROUD I am of you. You are an amazing young man. You are your own man. Someone I look up to in many ways. I am very proud to say you are my son.*

- *And last, what you are GOOD at. And you are not just good but great at being with people. You are a great friend and your major in the school of communication fit you well. At work you are good on the phone with the customers and also in your ability to handle the people that come into the office.*

Kirk, I am so proud of your grades this year. You just completed your best year in college. I know it brought your GPA up. Only a little more than a year to go to get your degree. Hang in there, you can do it, son.

I cannot believe it has been nine months since you proposed to the love of your life. In about three weeks you will be married. You have never lived anywhere else in your life. It just seems so strange. I am sure we will get used to it, but the house will not be the same without you living here. I want you to know that I believe you are ready for this move and you did a good job finding a place to live. Son, I pray that the two of you continue to keep the communication lines open and clear. Don't withhold anything from each other and never stop telling her how much you love and appreciate her. Never take her for granted.

Son, as you go on with your life as a husband, leader of your home, and someday father, I wish I had some great words of wisdom, but I don't. All I can say is to be yourself and love God. Keep him in the center of your home and always put your wife first in everything. I love working with you and I am always here for you. I am sure your relationship will change and I look forward to this new season in our relationship. I have a vision of us just hanging out together, and enjoying the gift you are.

I was really blessed when you asked your two brothers to be in your wedding. Kevin will make a great best man. I love the relationship you have with them and I can see you have a special place in your heart for them. I pray that your friendship lasts a lifetime. Enjoy the ride!

Son, you know how much I love you and I will support you in whatever you do.

Lastly, I want to tell you how much I enjoy the time we spend at work and our lunch talks. I look forward to many more lunches.

I love you very much and look forward to seeing you in your new roles and growing your new family.

May god bless you all the days of your life . . .

Dad

The Fourth Letter

October 22, 2005

Dear Mom and Dad,

A short time ago, a friend asked me whether I made an effort to pattern myself after any other person in my personal or business life. Since I have never been asked this question before, I thought of a few names of people I admire, but I told my friend that I don't believe I have consciously imitated any person's style or characteristics.

As I drove home after that conversation, I gave more thought to this question. Then the answer came to me in a flash.

If I could have possibly patterned myself after anyone, it would be both of you.

There are few people who are universally liked. All of us have at least a few negative traits that somehow offend others. But this is not the case with you. There is absolutely no one who does not like both of you. The reasons are obvious – you are genuine, caring and friendly people who manage to be admired by everyone you encounter.

Then there is your courage. I had a hard time moving from one part of town to another to another, but you brought your children thousands of miles to a foreign country with little help from others. When we found that our first stop was not suitable for us, instead of turning back, you did not hesitate in moving on to a better place.

I seriously doubt that I could have made a move to the United States with young children, no financial support and no assurances of employment.

Your positive spirit always taught us that anything can be accomplished. Whenever you faced an obstacle in the road, you did not dwell on the negatives. You simply found a way to remove that object or maneuver around it to reach your goal.

Then there is your sense of humor. When times were rough, you still managed to retain your humor. Dad enjoys a good joke, even when he happens to be the target of that joke. He may have heard the same joke countless times, but his face still reddens with laughter when he hears it again.

Your unselfish nature always directs both of you to think about the needs of others before you consider your own needs. All your efforts in life have been devoted to others, yet you never ask for or expect recognition for your good deeds.

You have faced hardships in life that would have easily broken others, but somehow, you have always gained strength from those adverse experiences. You became even more determined to improve the life of your family with each setback. You were never defeated and you never claimed to be victims. You taught us to maintain a deep sense of pride, despite adversities.

Even though you would not consider yourselves wealthy, you are actually the richest people I know because of your close-knit family and circle of friends who are completely devoted to you. How many can honestly say that they are truly happy with who they are and what they have accomplished in life? Yet, this is who you are – never asking or wanting for more.

From the moment we arrived in this country, you stressed the importance of education. You did everything possible to insure that every educational opportunity was available to us, even though it further strained your finances.

You engrained in us a strong sense of honor. You do not have the capacity to mislead others. Your word is your bond. You happen to be among that rare group who can honestly say that their integrity has never been questioned.

Your highest priority has always been family and friends above everything else. You came to this country for one reason, to provide your children with a better quality of life. You worked long hours for decades, often late at night and on weekends, because providing for them was always your goal.

Yet despite all the challenges you faced, I can't remember ever hearing either of you complain about the burdens placed on you.

You are sensitive and gentle souls who care about others, particularly those in need. You never ask for favors, but instead, you prefer to grant favors. You were the pioneers who encouraged many family members and friends to this country so they could also enjoy more opportunities. Your house was always a safe haven for those seeking comfort and support.

There were times that I am sure you may have disagreed with a path I took in life, but to your credit, you let me go my way. You always showed confidence in your children and supported our decisions. You guided us, but never tried to change us. Both of you sacrificed in every way to make our lives better. Most importantly, you always showed your love for us regardless of what we may have done.

I could work every minute of every day for the rest of my life, but I could not possibly even get close to enjoying the same treasure of good qualities as the two of you possess. This is because all these wonderful attributes come natural to you.

I am truly blessed that God chose me to be your son.

I love you more than you could possibly know.

On the following page is an email I would like to share sent to me by the author of this letter.

Hi Gayla,

Thank you for your suggestion to write a letter to a loved one before it is too late. After we spoke a couple of years ago, I think I mentioned that I attended a memorial service in which I honored a deceased friend. You know that I then sent a letter to my parents.

Yesterday was my dad's funeral. I took the opportunity to read excerpts of the letter to a "sold out" house in the chapel at the memorial park. I am so thankful that I had an opportunity to say these things to him before he passed on when it was more meaningful.

I cannot tell you how many people approached me during dinner to say that they were weeping as I read that letter. A number of them also said that they plan to do the same for a loved one.

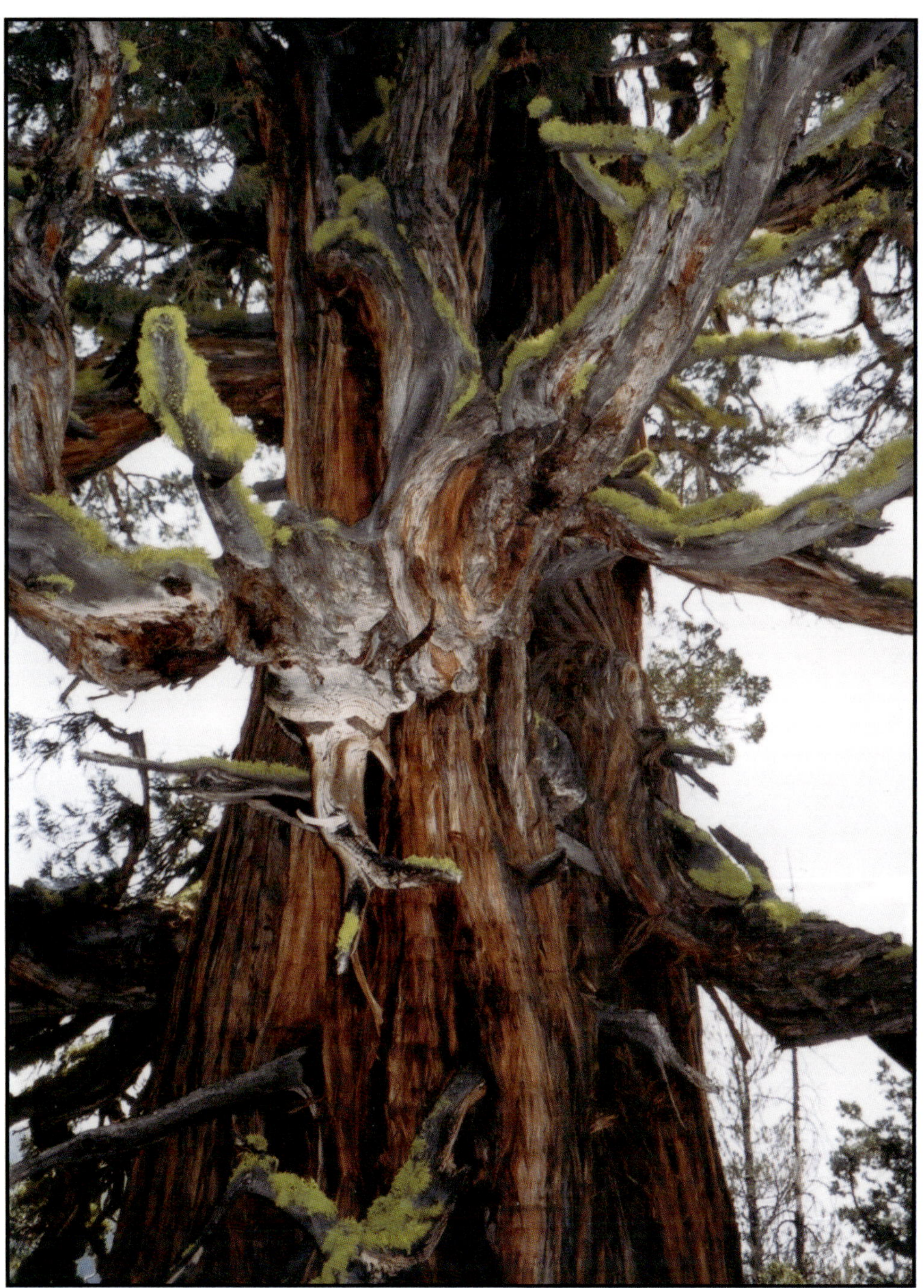

Photo by Gayla Gabriel

Gratitude

> **"A thankful heart is not only the greatest of virtues, but the parent of all other virtues."**
>
> ***Cicero, 106 BC – 43 BC***

Gratitude is a concept that can help us say thank you for the many experiences, both negative and positive, that we encounter during our lifetime. Acknowledging the effect of these personal experiences of love, success, growth, and happiness is one way we can express our gratitude. Expressing gratitude for the experiences in our lives that caused chaos or were not ones we liked can give us an appreciation for accepting the outcome or the growth we made during those challenging times. Gratitude allows us to see more fully that it is possible for negative experiences to be turned into positive experiences.

- Take some time to review past and present events in your life that have truly made you feel grateful.

- Perhaps there is a person who helped to add to your life in a monumental or even small way - thank them.

- Create a message that speaks of your gratitude. It may be a personal message for a special someone and/or a general message revealing more about yourself and your gratitude for the many things you have in your life.

- Creating a note of gratitude can start with a wonderful card or beautiful stationery upon which you write your message.

You might begin:

> I am grateful for all the years I have been your mother, wife, husband, or father . . .
>
> I am grateful for the many wonderful moments we shared as friends, or lovers . . .
>
> I feel full of gratitude for the many words of wisdom you shared with me throughout my life . . .

Place the completed notes in the envelope provided.

Appreciation

"Appreciation is an actual spiritual force,
a packet of energy that protects all that we hold dear in our hearts,
offering thanks is a tool for us to safeguard the joy and treasures we possess."

This exercise will awaken you to thinking about everyday things in your life that you appreciate. The list can include loved ones, family members, pets, the gifts of nature, certain moments of the day or those events that stand out in your memory. These are all the sparks of light in your life.

Think about the concept of appreciation. When something is appreciated it increases in value. When we lose something or someone in our lives our desire to have whatever it is back in our lives is heightened. We realize the complacency in our appreciation only when we are awakened to the pain of loss. Right now you have an opportunity to reflect on your present life and everything and everyone you value and cherish. Create a list of all things that are valuable to you and that you truly appreciate in your life. Then next to each one write a short statement about how its value steadily increased as your appreciation was realized.

This information will reveal a part of you that can be quite surprising.

I Appreciate . . .

I Appreciate . . .

What Do I Treasure?

There is a difference between appreciating and treasuring something or someone. When you appreciate something it becomes more valuable to you. It appreciates in value. A treasure is something that you love, enjoy, makes you feel good, and enhances your life. What are those things in your life that you treasure?

It's possible that a few of the treasures you name will also be written under the "I Appreciate" section, especially the names of people you love. Create the list knowing you are revealing precious jewels of information about yourself.

In the space provided make your list of treasures. Then sit back and reflect upon your feelings. Return to the list and write next to each one why it is a treasure.

List of Treasures . . .

List of Treasures . . .

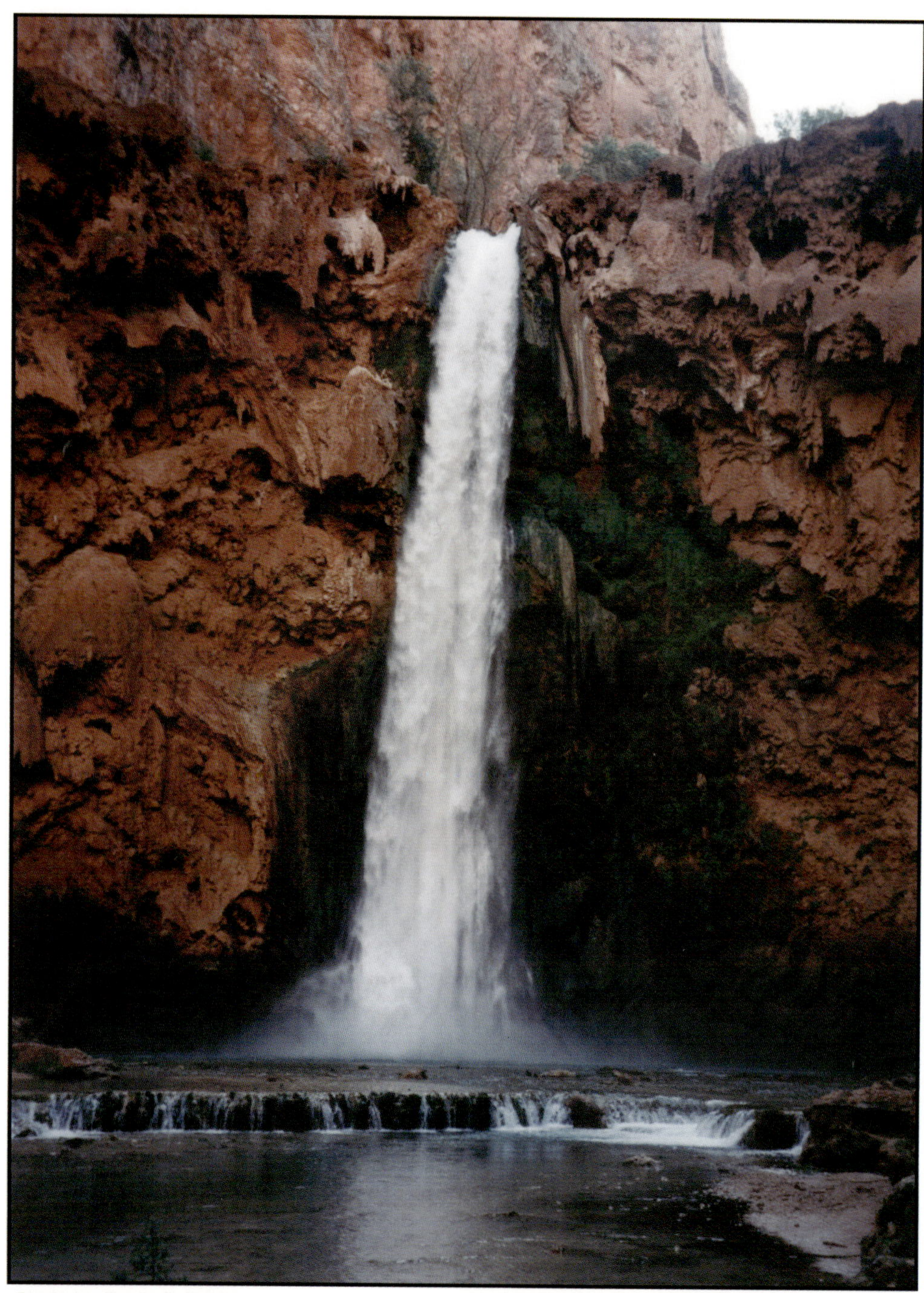

Photo by Gayla Gabriel

Gifts From My Heart

This exercise requires that you look through your personal belongings and reflect on which ones hold a special place in your memory or heart. It might be an item that was given to you by someone who has passed on, or maybe the person is still living. It could be you bought the item for yourself on a special occasion or it was a birthday or anniversary gift. These items may include jewelry, books, furniture, dishes, records, CDs, clothing, crystals, sacred objects, or sentimental memorabilia.

This exercise may take several days. Allow yourself the time to sit with these personal objects and reflect upon how you feel about each one. While involved in this process, you may have a thought about a loved one or friend. It's possible their name might pop into your head or you will see them in your mind's eye. You may even remember someone commenting on and admiring a particular item. Maybe they gave the item to you as a gift.

Create an inventory for these items by:

- Developing a written list of the objects.
- Photographing each item.

Now, using your inventory list or photographs of these objects, decide who will receive each one. Make a few notes including the name of the person the item will be given to upon your death and why.

- You might choose to be elaborate and wrap certain items like gifts.

Forgiveness & Forgiving

"Without forgiveness life is governed by an endless cycle of resentment and retaliation."

Roberto Assagioli, M.D., 1888 – 1974
Western Psychologist
Founder of Psychosynthesis

Frank Ostaseski, Founding Director of both the Zen Hospice Project, the first Buddhist Hospice in America created in San Francisco in 1987, and the Metta Institute, a training center for end-of-life care practitioners, caught my attention when he appeared on the Oprah Winfrey Show several years ago. He eloquently shared his personal experiences while sitting with people nearing the end of their lives and noted that the question, "Have I loved well?" was their main concern. After seeing this interview I enrolled in the profound and deeply moving, "Opening to Life Workshop Series" facilitated by Frank Ostaseski. During these workshops, Frank shared the importance of forgiveness and its transformative ability to restore one's confidence in our innate ability to love.

Is there someone you need forgiveness from or you need to forgive? Are you willing to explore and engage in the practice of forgiveness, by recognizing your need to ask someone for their forgiveness or to forgive? Here is an opportunity for creating a powerful and positive impact on your life. Consider composing a letter asking for or giving forgiveness. The writing of this letter will bring an incredible healing for you and the one receiving this message. Be challenged by your immediate response and allow yourself to be involved in this process. Remember that forgiving is not about approving negative

behavior, yours or someone else's. Put aside who was right or wrong. Just be in the moment of forgiving and perhaps being forgiven in return. This is a powerful act! It will clear unsettled energy between you and that other person, releasing old hurts, guilt, and resentment so you can restore that part of your life. Own your feelings, speak from a loving and caring place; none of us are perfect, but asking to be forgiven and forgiving can clear a space inside of your heart allowing you to leave with love.

In my grief counseling practice, one of the most important exercises a grieving client will do to help with his or her recovery is the writing of a letter to the person involved with the loss or experience they are grieving. The letter includes statements asking to be forgiven, or forgiving someone, apologizing, expressing their disappointments, or expressing their love. Again, writing these feelings on paper is powerful! After completing this process, my clients report feeling lighter, as if a heavy weight has been lifted from their shoulders.

I know you too will sense an opening or change deep inside yourself. The recipient of your letter may also experience a change. However, the most important part of this exercise is the healing you will initiate and create.

Notice your hesitation, put your ego aside and start this exercise.

There are many ways to start the process of forgiveness:

Select some beautiful music to help set the mood.

- Pause and reflect on what the circumstances were that led you to be angry, sad, disappointed, betrayed, abandoned, or resentful.
- What were you expecting or asking for that did not turn out the way you anticipated?
- Take time to reflect on the situation.
- Now see if in your heart of hearts you can put into words how you feel.
- Allow the music to help you engage with your emotions.
- Write those feelings on paper.
- Use compassion as you compose this note or letter asking forgiveness from the person you have been angry with or who has been angry with you all this time.
- Starting a note about forgiveness is often difficult. Here are a few suggestions:

  At this time I am asking for your forgiveness for . . .

  It is important to me that you know I forgive you for . . .

  It is my wish that you will forgive me for . . .

  Please forgive me for . . .

  I can now forgive myself for . . .

After composing the note:

- Fold it and put it away for a day or two.
- Take it out and reread it.
- If it feels right for you, seal it in an envelope addressed to the recipient, and put it in the envelope that has been provided.

- You are now creating a part of your keepsake.
- If the letter is for someone still living you may decide to deliver it personally sometime soon or arrange to have it delivered.

Be courageous and take the time to start writing this letter now.

If the letter is for someone that has died create a ceremony as simple as imagining them receiving your letter. One of my teachers once said that the soul of the person that has died receives the messages. Your letters may be buried, burned or torn up. Releasing any remnants of them into the wind or ocean can result in a wonderful feeling of letting go.

Store these messages in the following envelope.

Where Have I Been & Where Am I Going?

"Every day should be passed as though it were our last."

Publilius Syrus (-100 BC)

Where have you been and where are you going? What have you imparted to your loved ones, children, and friends? Are there values and beliefs that you have lived your life by and want to share with others? What are your hopes and dreams for your children individually or as a family? Writing sincere loving feelings will open your heart. As a result, your notes, letters or stories will reveal interesting information about you. All that you share will become a priceless gift for those receiving your messages.

Starting to write these notes, letters or stories will take time. Here are some ideas to help you begin:

- As I look back through the years of my life . . .
- I would like to share some of the most valuable lessons I learned during my life . . .
- Some of the most important events in my life were . . .
- Extraordinary occurrences I witnessed in my life that changed, broadened, saddened me were . . .

Place the completed notes in the envelope provided.

Meaningful Activities

What activities in life have been meaningful? Did you ever cook for bake sales to raise money, read to the blind, or cuddle sick babies in hospitals? Have you volunteered in a classroom assisting a teacher or helping the kids? Have you ever walked or run for one of the foundations that sponsored events for AIDS, cancer, leukemia, or another cause? Do you love playing the piano, dancing or painting? This would be a great time to share these personal activities and explain why each one is meaningful. Perhaps hiking or swimming in the ocean is meaningful to you. Whatever the activities are, share how they have been meaningful.

My Activities . . .

My Activities . . .

Revelations

"[Memory is] a man's real possession.
In nothing else is he rich, in nothing else is he poor."

Alexander Smith, 1830 – 1867
Scottish Essayist & Poet

What "aha" moments have touched your life and made a difference in something you have done? What epiphanies made you more vibrant? Share these experiences now. How wonderful for you to have had those moments! Recording your revelations on tape, DVD, or video would be an excellent way to make your story come alive.

Ideas for starting your story:

- One of the most amazing moments in my life that truly touched me and made a difference was the time when . . .
- Through life's experiences I have learned so many extraordinary things that I would like to share a few with you . . .
- I must share something magical that happened to me . . .

Place the completed notes in the envelope provided.

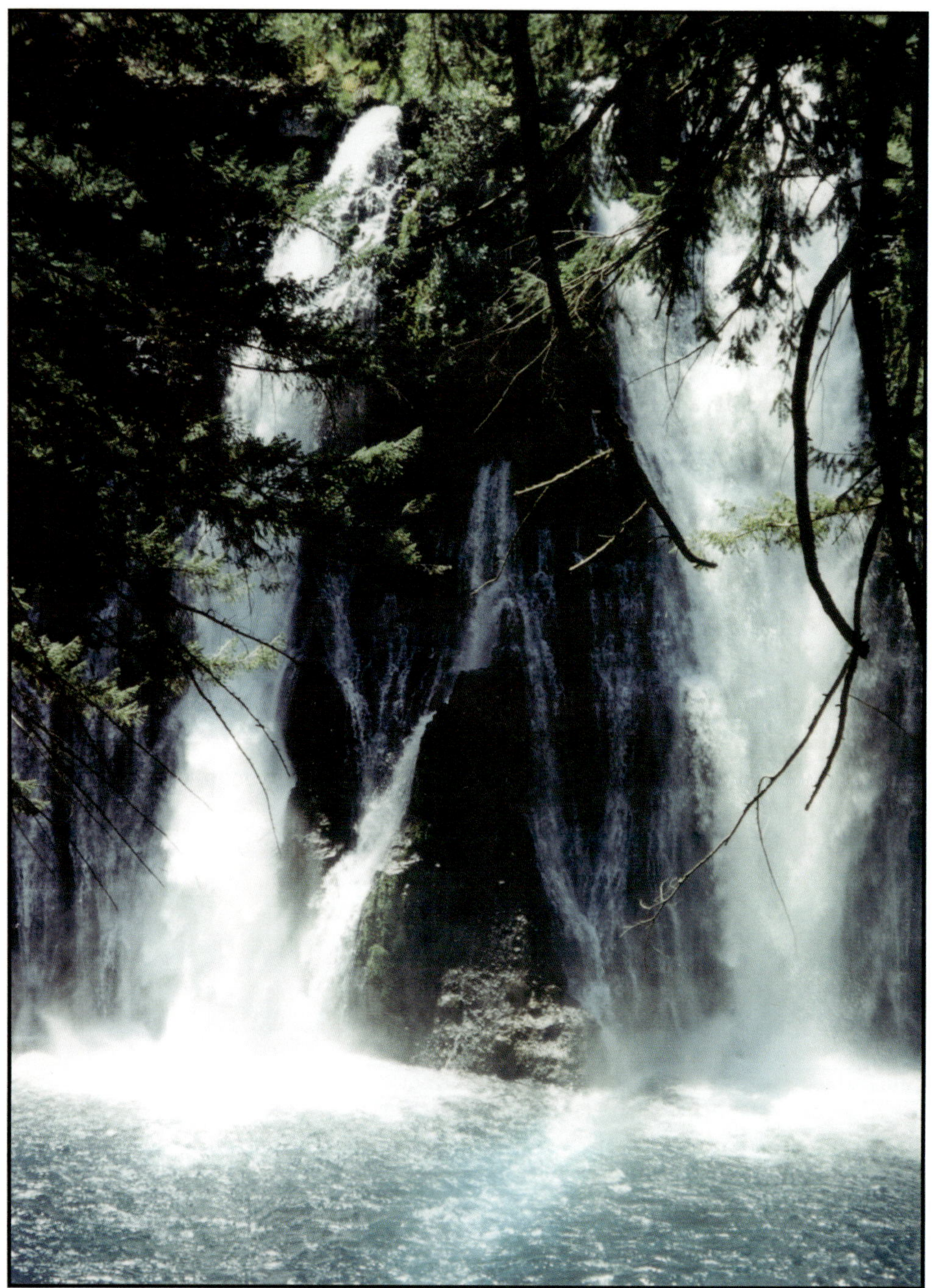

Photo by Gayla Gabriel

Moments That Warmed My Heart, Put A Smile On My Face & Brought Laughter From My Lips

In this world of so much seriousness we need to hold on to those precious moments that money cannot buy. Those times are priceless. Remember something you did as a child. Something valuable someone said to you. A moment created by one of your children that floods back into your memory as you are reading this sentence. Allow that warm and wonderful moment to wash over you, experiencing it again. Now keep that smile on your face and write about it as you share that precious moment, allowing it to flow onto the paper.

Moments – Smiles – Laughter

Moments – Smiles – Laughter

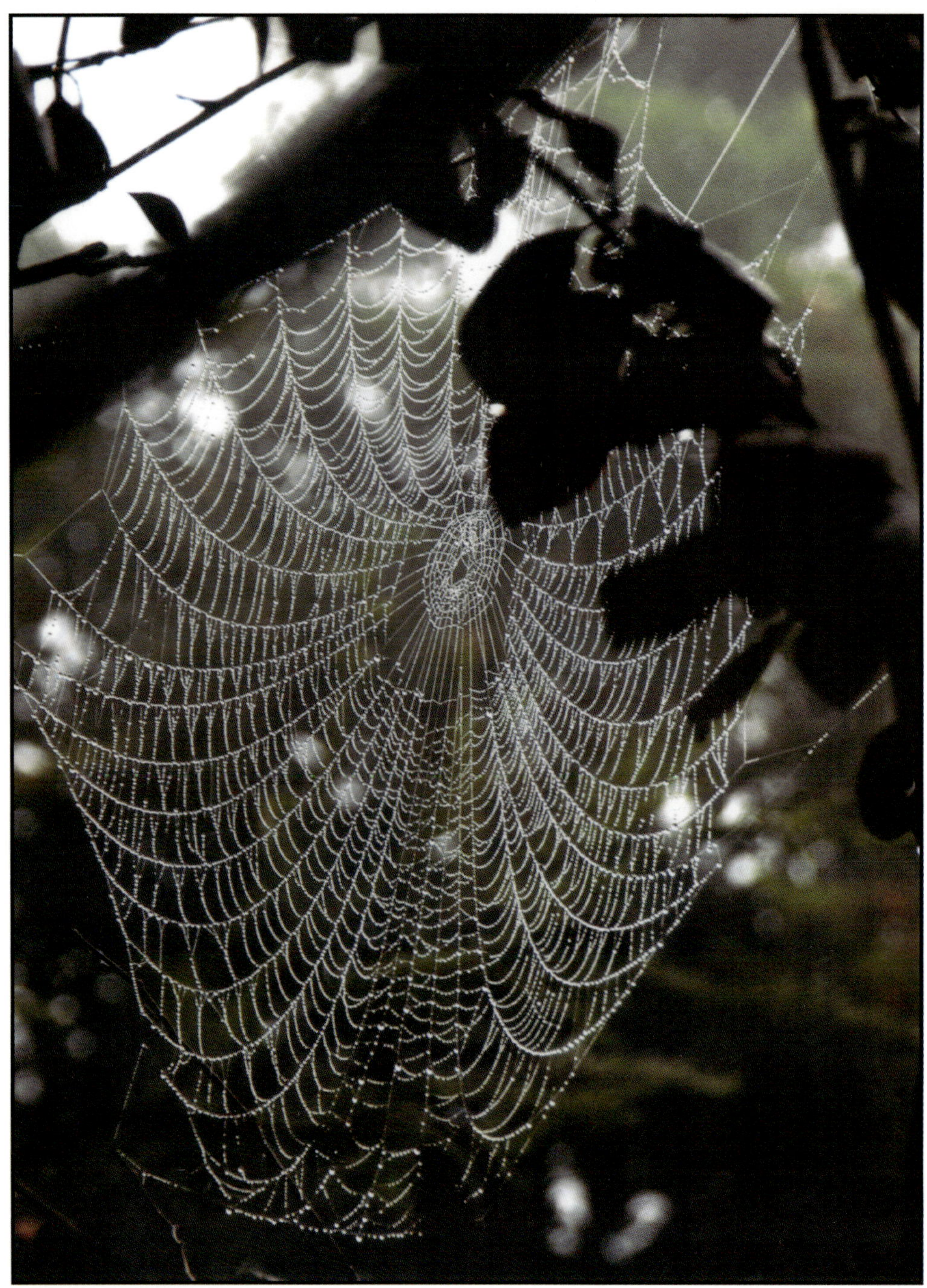

Photo by Janet Carnay

Regrets

Most of us either have no problem admitting to regrets we have or wish the regrets would go away. Most likely, we regret something we have done or something that we wish we might have accomplished in this lifetime. How many times do we hear ourselves saying that familiar phrase, I could've, would've, should've? Reflect on those moments or catch yourself when you are about to say I wish I would have.

There might be comical moments or situations that you experienced and wished you had done differently.

The regrets you choose to share will definitely reveal more about you and will be remembered.

Use the space below to write about some of these regrets and ponder the one or two you might do something about now.

You might begin by saying:

- I would like to share with you some things I regret having done in my life . . .
- My hopes are that after you read about some of my regrets you will more fully understand the complexity of my life . . .

My Regrets . . .

My Regrets . . .

My Favorite Books

"Books are the quietest and most constant friends;
they are the most accessible and wisest of counselors,
and the most patient of teachers."

Charles W. Eliot – The Happy Life, 1896

Compiling a list of some of your favorite books is an opportunity to share what you have enjoyed with friends and loved ones. Take inventory of these books and then make a list of the titles. After the title of each book listed, write the name of the person you would like to give the book to as a gift. You might even inscribe a special note inside the book to the person receiving it. Maybe you can even give it to them now. Repeating this process with your favorite music, films or photos can also be done at this time.

My Favorite Books . . .

My Favorite Books . . .

Leaving My Pets With Love

Do you have pets that you love? If you do then you know that they have feelings. They will miss you and need to be cared for and loved upon your death. Talk about this with family and friends as a "what if" to get a feeling about who would like to or be able to take care of your best friend or feline. Consider whom they would be happiest with if you were not there to take care of them. Choose someone special to leave them with in case of your death. You might also consider leaving money for the welfare of your pet if your budget permits. Of course, leaving money might require a will or legal document. This money might come in handy during their adjustment period. Your pet's name, his vital information, a list of his/her favorite foods and their veterinarian is necessary for a smooth transition. Filling out the following page will help pass on this vital information.

About My Pet

NAME

____

PERSON TO INHERIT PET & PHONE NUMBER

____

VETERINARIAN'S NAME & PHONE NUMBER

____

GROOMER'S NAME & PHONE NUMBER

____

FAVORITE FOODS

____

BIRTHDAY OR AGE

____

SPECIAL INFORMATION ABOUT MY PET

____

____

____

____

____

____

SPECIAL INFORMATION CONTINUED

About My Pet

NAME

____

PERSON TO INHERIT PET & PHONE NUMBER

____

VETERINARIAN'S NAME & PHONE NUMBER

____

GROOMER'S NAME & PHONE NUMBER

____

FAVORITE FOODS

____

BIRTHDAY OR AGE

____

SPECIAL INFORMATION ABOUT MY PET

____

____

____

____

____

____

SPECIAL INFORMATION CONTINUED

Blessings I Would Like To Leave For Those I Love

"As you prepare this beautiful keepsake filled with personal eternal messages, may you be blessed and become immortal through the love you are sharing."

Gayla Gabriel – Author

Think of one of your favorite blessings or make up one with the idea of communicating a wonderful message to someone you love. Blessings come from love and the desire to convey your intention to wish someone love, happiness, sustenance, healthy children, recovery from an illness, or any other sentiment of hope. Blessings and good intentions can also be created for a new home, building, boat, car or whatever you think warrants more positive energy.

Be creative! Think about those you love and what is going on in their lives that could use your connecting them to the energy of a source greater than all of us. A blessing has the ability to send this message.

When you have finished creating your blessings, personalize each one and place them in the envelope provided or share them now.

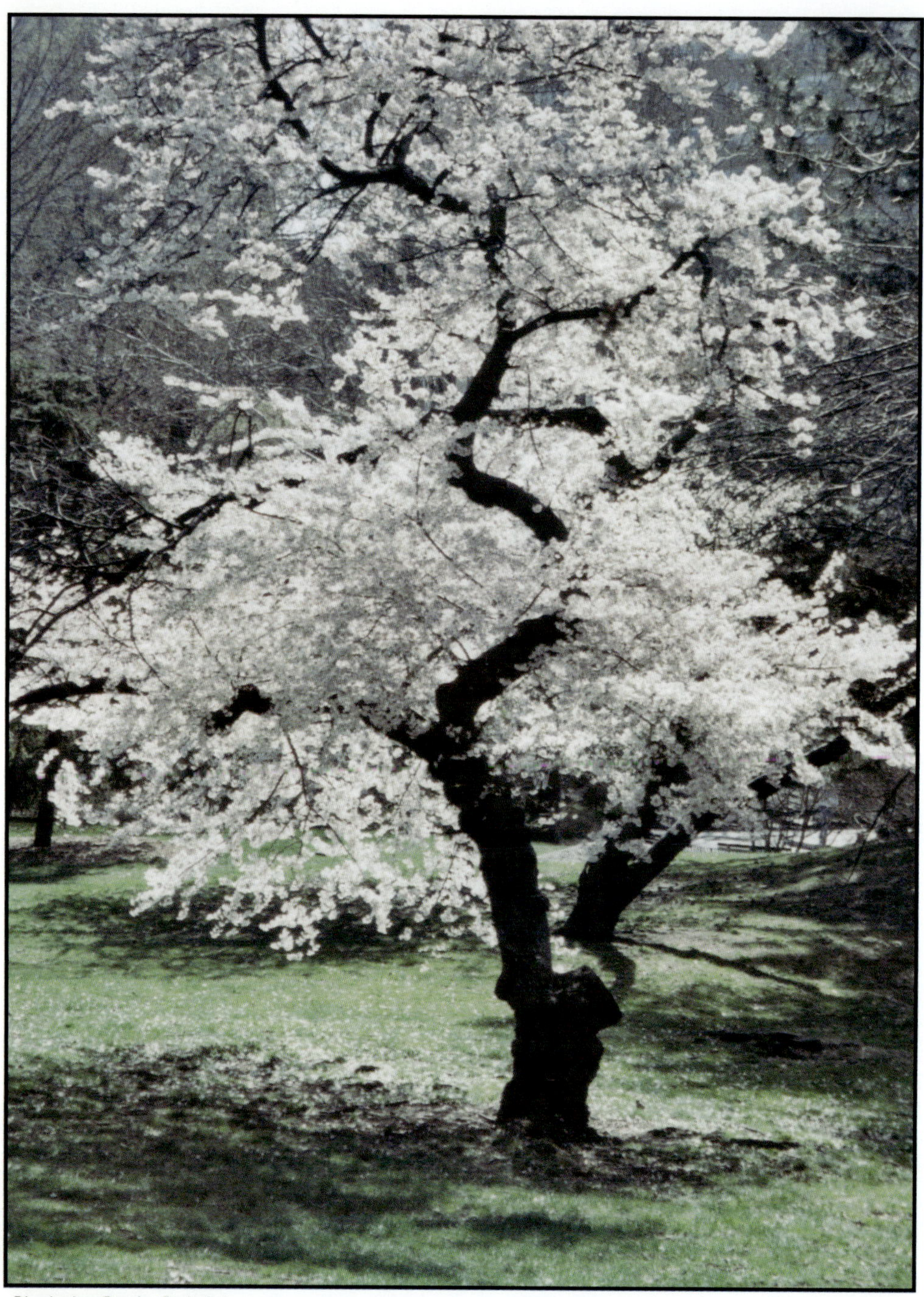

Photo by Gayla Gabriel

Planning My Funeral

"Neither the sun nor death can be looked fully in the face."

Francois de la Rochefoucauld, 1613-1680

In our society today we plan for the birth of a baby, celebrate certain designated birthdays, confirmations, christenings, bar and bat mitzvahs, engagements, weddings, and so on. However, when it comes to planning our own death, which is a certainty, we become death-denying and do not want to discuss the subject. We have difficulty facing the impermanence of our physical life and everything as we know it. If you are not facing a life-threatening illness at this time you probably feel this planning is premature and depressing. Nonetheless, it would be pertinent for us to remember that none of us know for sure when we will breathe our last breath. We have witnessed 9/11 that left hundreds of unsaid good-byes, and most of us have had the personal experience of losing or hearing about the unexpected death of someone by accident or heart attack. For instance, the deaths of Princess Diana and John F. Kennedy, Jr. were totally unexpected. You can probably think of many people who died unexpectedly and realize we are all vulnerable to death.

Planning your own funeral is a process that can be a relief both for you and those you leave behind. Your family will be grateful and relieved that they have been left with your personal plan. Leaving a plan that includes your wishes and requests for your funeral will allow this ceremony to reflect your clear intentions.

Now is the time to consciously plan for your death by making decisions about how your last rites will be handled. There are many decisions to be made by you alone or together with your loved ones. Recording these decisions will relieve those that love you from feeling they missed something you might have wanted at your funeral, memorial service, or wake.

One way to begin the planning is to do a short meditation. Create a 20-30 minute pause in your life for this quiet time without the interruptions of family, phone, TV, or other distractions. Then enlist the help of some beautiful music - may I suggest a few titles: Graceful Passages - Gary Remal Malkin (use the CD without the messages for this exercise), Beyond the Horizon - Hilary Stagg (or any of his CD's), or The Music of the Grand Canyon - Nicholas Gunn, just to name a few.

Find a comfortable place to sit, turn the music on, relax, take a deep cleansing breath and close your eyes. Now take another deep breath, allow the music in and follow your breath. Imagine you have left this world, passed on, and you are watching your funeral from another time and space. What is the mood? Where is it? How many people are there? Do you hear another track of music? Are people speaking about your life? Are poems or passages from the Bible or some other book being read? Do you see a favorite priest, rabbi, or another spiritual practitioner? What do the surroundings look like? Are there flowers, plants, mountains, an ocean, or a river?

Imagine how you would like those attending to feel. Notice your own feelings, stay present and allow it to feel real just for now. Sit with this image as you arrange in your mind's eye all the details that would please you and your loved ones. When you are OK with what you have created slowly move farther above the setting until you no longer can see the details. Take a deep breath and slowly open your eyes. Now for a few moments reflect on your meditation.

Are you ready to write down some of the details that will help plan that ceremony you just visited in your meditation? The following is a list you could fill in for the planning of your funeral to aid those you leave behind.

Funeral Planning List

Burial or cremation? ______________________

Do you already have a burial plot? ______________________

Do you have a plan paid for at a particular cemetery?

____

Where and at what cemetery would you like to rest?

____

Coffin or urn? ____________ Type of coffin or urn? ____________

Name of the person(s) who will lead the service and their contact information:

____

Type of service? Graveside, chapel, memorial, roast, other:

____

Favorite flowers: ______________________

Charitable donations? ______________________

Favorite charities: ______________________

Favorite scriptural passages:

____

Music to be played:

Poems to be read:

Eulogy to be given by:

Your own message to be read:

Special foods to be served:

Wishes:

Pallbearers or ushers:

People To Be Notified

(This list will change over time. If you have an alternate list on your cell phone, you have highlighted names in an address book, or you have created an email list, note the information here.)

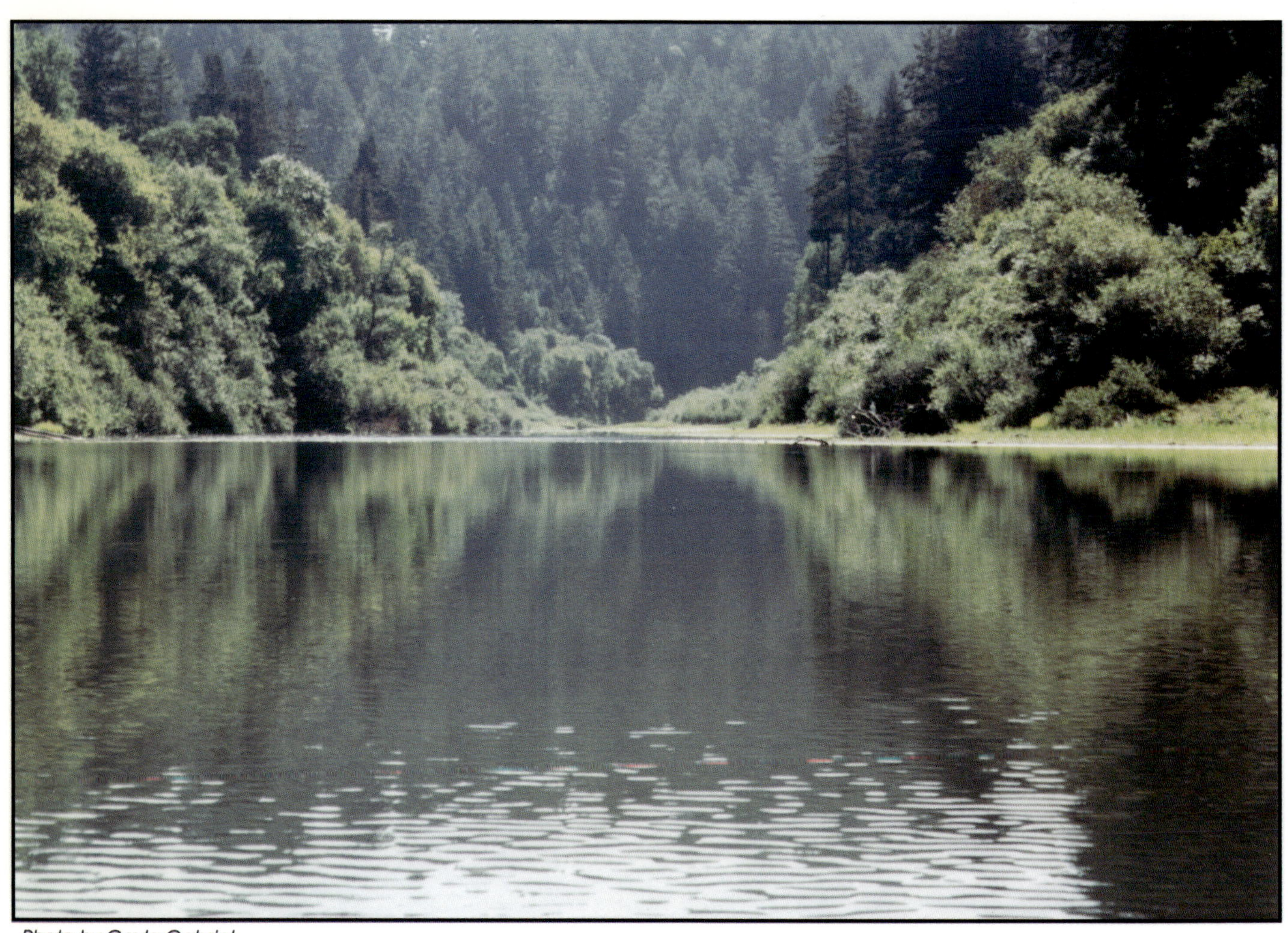

Photo by Gayla Gabriel

Writing My Obituary

"A life unexamined is not worth living."
Socrates, 470 BC – 399 BC

Here is an opportunity to create your own obituary. This may seem strange; however, this is a way to insure that all the information about you is correctly written. Look in your daily newspaper and review the details of some of the obituaries. You will notice short ones and fairly lengthy ones. Perhaps you might use the longer example of an obituary that you find interesting to model your own. You might want to do it in pencil, because the information may change over the years.

There is also the option of being creative. You might design a death announcement to be sent out after your passing to family and friends. This might be designed by you or a graphic artist. It could be a small card with a sketch of your likeness, your birth date, and something in the background like your favorite color, flowers, or on the back of it a favorite poem or some of your accomplishments. This is a touching and wonderful way for your loved ones to inform other family and friends of your passing. The announcement could also be used as a thank-you note acknowledging flowers, charitable donations, or someone's support.

Place the completed announcement and obituary in the envelope provided.

My Eulogy

Yes, you are being asked to write your own eulogy.

Writing your own eulogy is another gift for those you love. Of course, your loved ones might want to share their own thoughts about you, too. They can do that. However, composing your own eulogy is a beautiful and touching means of sharing important information about yourself. It's a review of the personal imprint you are leaving on the world. Throughout this book you have been asked to complete many exercises that you can refer to when composing your personal eulogy. Here's a list of some of the subjects you wrote about: your favorite things, regrets, special moments, revelations, things you would like to impart, personal treasures, appreciation, gratitude and forgiveness. Review some of these exercises and then make time to lovingly write about yourself. What has been said about you over the years and what important messages, images, feelings, and thoughts do you want to leave for your loved ones that will one day be gathered in your honor to say good-bye?

There's no right or wrong way to do this. Allow yourself the freedom to say whatever you want in your own special way. You might be funny, glib, serious, sentimental, or whatever else, but allow it to come from your heart.

Start it now...set the mood...play music...take yourself on a hike...go to the beach...the mountains...sit in your favorite chair. Imagine your funeral, the one you planned a few exercises before this one. See the place, those present, and the person you have asked to read your eulogy, clearing his or her throat and reading your personally composed eulogy.

Who is that person?

Write their name here and leave a note in the envelope asking them to please read your eulogy (you might ask a second person just in case one of them cannot do it).

Names:

____

____

____

Use your own stationery or paper to write the eulogy. Place the completed eulogy in the envelope provided.